The Morning Sickness Handbook

By Wendy Shaw

"A great joy
is
coming."

Disclaimer: *None of the information or products in this book are designed or implied to treat, diagnose or take the place of being under the care of a qualified medical doctor. Information found here represents my personal experiences, or that of others, and are here for your benefit in information, encouragement and support. Please make sure you stay in contact with a qualified health care professional.*

Photography by Holly Shaw
Cover Design by Chase Shaw

I thank the LORD for my husband, Kevin, and our blessings
Chase, Holly, Macy, Justus, Elley, Amy, Lilly, Peter,
Daniel and Joshua

I love you,

Mom

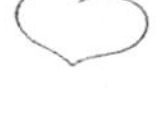

"Being a mother means
that your heart
is no longer yours;
it wanders wherever
your children do."

—Author Unknown

Table of Contents

....

Index:

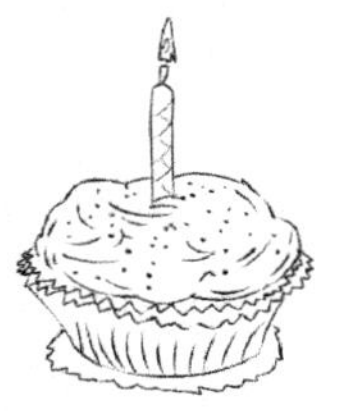

"Life is a flame that is
always burning itself out,
but it catches fire again
every time a child is born."

—George Bernard Shaw

Introduction

Congratulations on your pregnancy. You are blessed!

Nausea is common in pregnancy and means everything is going well! It's reported that over 80% of women experience some degree of it. And, although, it may have been keeping you from feeling as blessed as you should, there are many ways you can learn to use to overcome that nausea feeling.

Throughout my eleven pregnancies, I've learned a lot about the nature of nausea. There is no easy answer that fits everyone. It must be dealt with each day. But, once you know some easy tips and have the right resources, you can face it head on and win!

Women who have good support and solid information have a better chance of achieving much needed relief. Now you can discover a treasure of resources that many women have used for hundreds of years to overcome nausea.

Browse through more than 100 remedies and learn the strategies for success in using them.

"Success supposes endeavor."

–Jane Austen

Chapter 1

Morning Sickness Basics

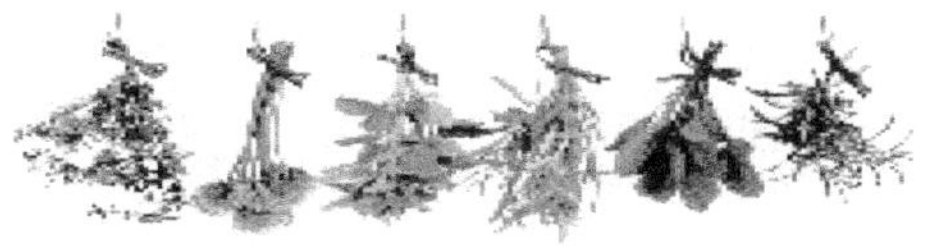

"I'm not afraid of storms, for I'm learning to sail my ship."

- Louisa May Alcott

There is no friendship,

no love,

like that of a mother

for her child.

–Henry Ward Beecher

Morning, Afternoon, and Evening Sickness.....

Morning Sickness should be renamed. Morning sickness is not just in the mornings. It can appear at any time of the day. If it does happen first thing in the morning, it doesn't always subside just because the afternoon is approaching. In fact, for many, nausea starts in the late afternoon, and lasts through the night. Nausea can show itself at anytime, coming and going, and sometimes, seemingly out of no where.

Morning Sickness is not a sickness, but a condition. An estimated 80% of pregnant women experience some degree of nausea discomfort in their pregnancy. It is not an indication that things are going wrong. Ironically, it means everything is going very right. Your hormones are kicking into gear and responding to nurture your growing baby.

How Long Will it Last?

On the extreme side, morning sickness can begin as early as 2 weeks and stop as late as after labor ends. But, these cases are more rare. Typically, nausea will begin anywhere between 4-6 weeks, peak between 8-9 weeks, and subside after week 13. However, It is not uncommon for women to have continued nausea through weeks 14-16, usually subsiding close to week 20.

COMMON MISCONCEPTIONS ABOUT PREGNANT MOMS:

.... They don't struggle with nausea if they are accomplishing their usual routines.

...It's always Ok for her to talk about/fix/smell food.

...She looks great, so she must feel great, too!

Why?

No one knows for sure! Your HCG (human chorionic gonadotropin) hormone may play a role. Other active hormones are progesterone, estrogen, and cholecystokinin (increases digestion efficiency). Your baby's organ development is at its height from the 6th – 18th week. Your baby's rapid growth coupled with your hormone surge may be the culprit.

Some say the morning sick mom has too many toxins in her system (from an over-taxed liver) and that may cause it. Then there is the protein premise, the blood-sugar level connection, and more… there are many theories as to why nausea occurs. An interesting fact is, by the end of the third month, when the blood level of some of these hormones, levels off or starts to decline, in most cases, it seems to parallel the decrease in queasiness.

Most likely, you won't find the following statement headlining web sites selling nausea remedies: "*There is no absolute guaranteed cure.*" Until an airtight, across the board, solid, definitive reason is discovered for why morning sickness occurs, a one size fits all cure is difficult to promote. However, don't let this discourage you. Having proper info, support and strategies can go a long way to provide relief.

"To the world

you might just be one person,

But to one person

you might just be the world."

–Unknown

Chapter 2

Preparing for Success

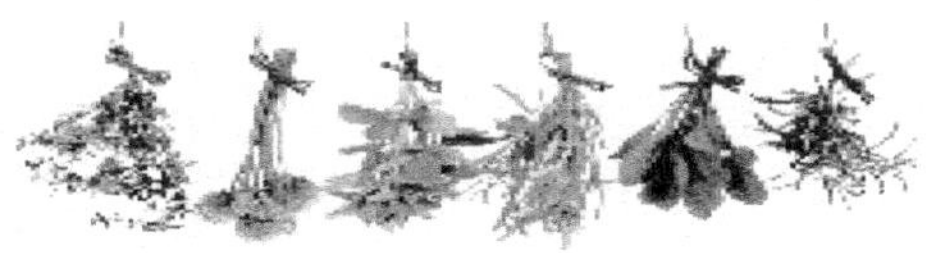

"Dwell in possibility."
-Emily Dickinson

Encouragement for Nauseous Moms

- Nausea really will end.

- You are doing a fantastic job of being a mom already.

- The amazing gift of life you'll meet is worth any challenges.

- You can do it!

"Children make your life important."

–Erma Bombeck

The Reality of Remedies

The wonderful thing about remedies is that women are all finding relief in different ways. This gives much hope to those who find their friend's advice didn't work for them. Women are still able to find their own helpful remedy.

Whatever your remedy of choice is, it is not a forever cure. Nausea will keep coming back and you will need to stay on top of it. For most women, as the pregnancy progresses, the times needed to think about it, become less and less. And, for some, you can do so well preventing it, that you may never be bothered by it, again.

Things to remember: Your chosen remedy may not seem consistent. Some "cures" can help in the morning, but not in the afternoon, or only in the evening, etc.. They can stop working, when they previously were, and then start to work again without predictability. That doesn't mean it's a "dud," only it's just one item in your complete remedy line-up. If something doesn't help now, but used to,…. Keep trying. It may just need to be reintroduced at a later time, or alongside a different remedy.

Each remedy is as unique as the woman who is experiencing the nasuea. What works for one person, might not work for someone else. Why? Because your body has its own biorhythms, stress levels, nutrition and exercise routines, toxin levels and hormone dynamics that will fluctuate as the pregnancy progresses. All this influences the effectiveness of any remedy combination. Your choice may be entirely different than what worked for your friend. What I, or anyone else can do, is offer you suggestions, tips and advice so that you can make the best educated decision possible. You know yourself best!

Our natural body rhythms and hormones change as the pregnancy progresses. As you find yourself gravitating towards a few specific remedies, start with these in combinations or singularly, but be ready to switch out as needed. Experiment with new ideas, go back to old standbys, it's all about finding what your body needs at that moment. Don't give up hope. If you can't seem to find the right thing at first, it may just mean you need to put different remedy combos together.

I'll introduce you to preconception strategies first (for next time) and then the overall Top10 Remedies. You can skip this part and go to the next section, if you prefer. There you will read about remedies you probably have in your kitchen right now. Then you can dive into the A-Z resource and pick out more of your soon to be favorites!

Preconception Preparation

3-6 months or more before conception.

These suggestions are good for every season of our lives!

1) **Eat healthy.** Cut out excess fats and sugars. Consume raw fruits, vegetables, nuts, and seeds. Eat foods that are most closely to their natural state. I recommend good books to read in Part 5, Resource section.

2) **Get regular exercise.** The process of carrying a child for nine months , including labor, can be very taxing on the body. The better condition your body can be in physically now, will give much benefit !

3) **Cleanse and detoxify.** Drink lots of water. Squeeze lemon or ACV in it for enhanced effect. Entrox or milk thistle, in particular are supplements recommended to help detoxify the liver and aid in digestion. There are many programs to choose from. See the Resource section for options.

4) Make sure you are taking a good **nutritional supplement.** Even food in its natural state could be missing many important nutrients because of soil conditions and other environmental factors. See Resources for Supplements.

5) **Supplement with Magnesium.** Liquid would be best. Magnesium needs to be stored up in our system. It helps us absorb vitamin b and zinc. Vitamin b is known to help curb nausea.

6) **Get Vitamin D naturally from sunlight.** 5 to 30 minutes of exposure to the skin on your face, arms, back or legs (without sun-screen) 2 times/week.

"In my belly for nine months,

in my heart forever."

-Unknown

THE TOP 10 FOR EVERYONE

1- Suck on crushed ice. Make your own ice cubes out of Kombu cha, Fruit Juice, Pregnancy tea, etc. Blend the ice to have the consistency of snow. Or, blend the liquid with ice. Use a small plastic spoon to eat it if you have a metallic taste in your mouth. Use pure water. Make sure the water you are using is not chlorinated or flouridated.

2- Lemon Aromatherapy. Keep lemon slices with you, or put the essential oil lemongrass on a damp washcloth, keeping it close at hand to bring to your nose when needed. Breathe slow and deep, focusing on a horizontal cue.

3- Wear loose fitting clothing around your waist. This will decrease the pressure on your already sensitive abdomen.

4- Move slow, when nauseous, especially your head. When rising, and with any movement., think SLOW!

5- Always keep something in your stomach. I know, it's a lot of work!! You're hungry, but the food won't stay down.
You want to eat, but gag at the thought of food. Keep trying...

(continued on next page)

...even though you don't feel any improvement, at first. Keep it small. (Avoid drinking liquid at the same time).

6- Try children's chewable vitamins when your prenatal vitamins are making you sick or you can't swallow them.

7- Easy, quick foods: Baby food, frozen fruit, granola bars, trail mix. Remember, with all food and drink, take small amounts, slowly letting each bite dissolve in your mouth before swallow ing. No matter how hungry you feel, chew thoroughly.

8- Eliminate odors and avoid places that have strong smells. (This on you probably figured out soon!) Fresh air is necessary. Keep windows open to capture fresh air, if you can. A personal fan with a combination of aromatherapy aimed directly at your nose can help.

9- Use Distractions. Whatever can help you get your mind off how miserable you are feeling: talking on the phone, shopping, driving, and watching a movie.

10- Keep your feet anchored. Whether lying down or sitting up, you must give your feet something to press against. (Keeps a sense of balance). If in bed, use the headboard.

Kitchen Remedies

Some things you may already have on hand that can be used!

Lemons
Fruit
Bananas
Bland Foods
Apple Cider Vinegar
Ginger
Ice
Molasses
Nuts
Beans
Olives
Peppermint candy
Popsicles
Herbal tea
Broth
Yogurt, kombucha, and other fermented foods

Read Chapter 3 for suggestions on how to use these common kitchen items to help overcome nausea.

"My mother was the most beautiful woman I ever saw. All I am I owe to my mother. I attribute all my success in life to the moral, intellectual and physical education I received from her."

– George Washington

Chapter 3

100 + Remedies for Relief

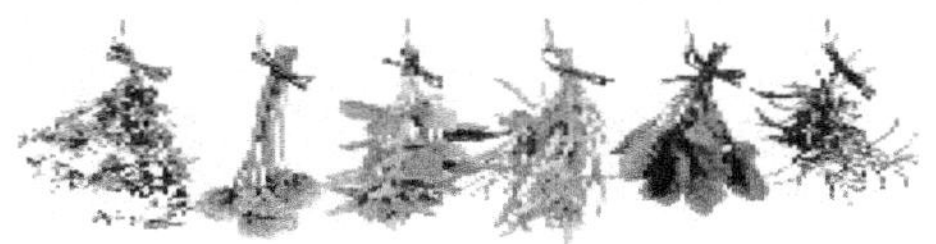

"A mother's joy begins when new life is stirring inside...
when a tiny heartbeat is heard for the very first time,
and a playful kick reminds her that she is never alone."

- Author Unknown

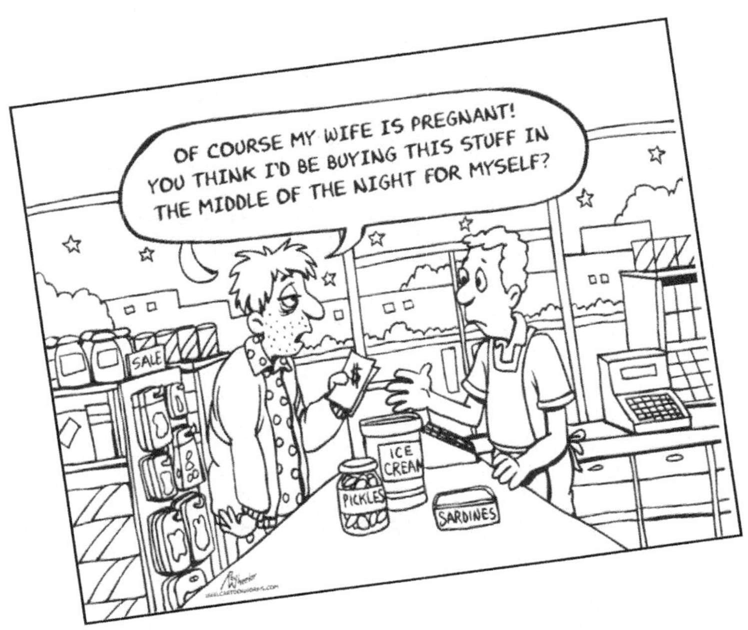
OF COURSE MY WIFE IS PREGNANT!
YOU THINK I'D BE BUYING THIS STUFF IN
THE MIDDLE OF THE NIGHT FOR MYSELF?
SALE
ICE CREAM
PICKLES
SARDINES

Your A-Z Remedy Guide

The first recorded episode of pregnancy nausea was 4,000 years ago. There are still many unanswered questions as to why it occurs, so there is no sure cure. Yet, while thinking of enduring nausea is not something anyone wants to do, be assured that relief is not outside of your grasp. Provided for you are over 100 remedy suggestions. This A-Z Remedy Guide is everything I have researched over the last 20 years. Find those things that sound good to you. Rotate and combine them. Remember any nausea remedy is not "one and done." You will need to stay on top of it. Think of any brief period of relief as a HUGE success!

What have you tried up until now?

-A-

Activated Charcoal. Mixed with water, sip slowly. Don't have within 2 hours of taking other supplements.

Acupuncture. Many women have said acupuncture reduced their nausea after a few sessions.

Acupressure. Daily overall massage is best. Both Eastern and Western medical practitioners describe the acupressure points that control nausea as the pressure point about 2 inches above the crease of the inner wrist. The two other points are in line with the little finger, and in the hollow between the collarbones. Press deeply and rub on these points for 5-7 seconds at a time, throughout the day. This is best when used in combination with other remedies. My sea bands became a permanent apparel item for me in some pregnancies. Make sure to choose a practitioner who brings only healthy spiritual aspects into their practice.

Acustimulation is a variation of acupressure which uses electrical stimulation. Has been found to reduce nausea in clinical studies. Use under attention of health care provider.

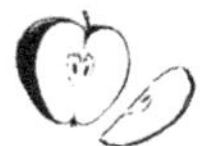

Apple Cider Vinegar. ACV can restore you ph balance. Put the vinegar in bath water (I cup) to absorb through skin, or mix with one ts per 8 ounces of purified drinking water to sip throughout the day. Or 1Tb ACV with 1 Tb honey in warm water first thing in the morning. Sip slowly. Make sure it is unfiltered with the "mother" in it. (Bragg.com)

Aromatherapy. Lemongrass, peppermint, lavender....Attach a hankie, that has essential oils on it, to a small personal fan. Warning! Don't try this with any synthetic smells. Use top quality essential oils, such as from Tropical Traditions, Young Living or DoTerra. *I used the essential oil lemongrass on a handkerchief and inhaled slowly and deeply, for several minutes until the feeling went away.*

Availability. Sometimes a food item is needed NOW!... Keep a small fridge or ice chest next to your bed. Then you don't have to walk or exert much effort to retrieve it. Consider having a kind person on standby in case you need something from the store and can't get it yourself.

Avoidance. Avoid..

- Smells, sights, sounds, that you find trigger nausea.
- Greasy, spicy, and fatty foods, unless absolutely craving them.
- Mixing solids and liquids in the same meal (wait 30 min-1 hr.).
- Negative people, this can add unnecessary stress.
- Fatigue - get lots of rest!

– B –

B-6, whole B, B-12. Researchers have found that pregnant women who take between 10 and 25 milligrams every eight hours get varying degrees of relief from their morning sickness. One study says that relief is within the first few doses, another states it must be taken 200 mg/day for a week to see the effects. Foods that contain Vitamin B naturally are: nutritional yeast, yogurt, bee pollen, spirulina, wheat germ, whole grains, egg yolk, cabbage and organically raised organ meats.

Important! Vitamin B must be absorbed to help. To help ensure it is utilized, take with Vitamin C. Whole food supplement are best. Liquid B is more easily absorbed.

Baby Food. The small jars of plums, bananas, or apricots are compact, ready to go, and easily available to provide convenient fruit intake.

Bananas. Slice & Freeze. Blend in smoothie.

Barley Water. Pour off the water used to cook barley, strain and drink. It balances your blood sugar and can resupply your energy level.

Baths. Your body absorbs water from a warm bath, and can help to rehydrate your system. Put ACV (1 cup) into the water to help balance ph levels, or put a few drops of essential oil (lavender or lemongrass) to help soothe you.

Beans. At the first hint of nausea, take 2-4 tablespoons of any cooked legume. You may need to repeat every 20 min - 4 hours. For the why this works details, visit: karenhurd.com

Beet Kvass- Purported for use as a digestive aid, blood tonic, liver cleanse and more. Take 3 medium organic beets chopped coarsely, add ¼ cup whey, 1 TB sea salt to a 2 quart container of filtered water. Put a lid on it and let it sit on the counter for 48 hours. Strain & consume.. *(Found in Nourishing Traditions by Sally Fallon (P.. 610))*

Bentonite Clay. This absorbs toxins in your stomach. Some have found taking this in the morning helped get them through the day. Mix I Tb. in juice or water.

Betaine HCI. This can allay nausea. If you feel bloated or queasy after eating protein foods, or you crave sour foods, than you may be deficient in hydrochloric acid. The suggested dose is 1-4 tablets with each meal. Begin with one tablet, and if you experience discomfort (an irritated stomach) cut back or stop.

Bland Foods. Potatoes, oatmeal, crackers, dry toast, dry cereal (Cheerios), rice, rice cakes, pasta, etc. ...neutral foods non-upsetting to stomach. Make sure to eat slow, small bites, really chewing well.

Bone Broth - ..from pasture raised beef is incredibly nutritious for your body. Keep in a crockpot and sip throughout the day. Season to taste.

Brewer's Yeast. For b6 and magnesium. It's also probiotic. Daily is best.

– C –

Calcium. If you take a calcium/magnesium supplement each day, it should help curb the sick feeling. Calcium must be taken with Magnesium as a 2 to1 ratio (for example: 1000 milligrams of Calcium/ 500 milligrams of Magnesium). Magnesium helps your body absorb the calcium. Chewable or fizzy calcium are 2 ways to take it. It is said that if taken before bed, it may neutralize stomach acids better.

Candy. Hard candy has helped many women. Sour candy, Jolly Ranchers, Lemon Heads. Remember to brush your teeth afterward., of course. *Organic sources are listed in the back.*

Chiropractor. Keep your body in optimum health & balance by including chiropractic care in your preventative health plan.

Chlorella. Lots of health in a small amount. Mix with water or juice.

Chlorophyll. 1 tablespoon per 8 oz. glass of water. For micronutrients.

Cleansing. Is nausea from built up toxins in your system? I highly recommend cleansing before pregnancy as it does aid your liver in fighting off any present toxins.

Coconut Oil. Therapeutic dose 2-3 Tbsp./day. Mix in with something else or let it dissolve in your mouth a little at a time. Drizzle or spread on anything and everything. (Read, "Coconut Cures," by Bruce Fife). *I LOVE this!*

Cola Syrup, Coca-Cola. Some women take this to feel better. You may want to try it as a cold slushy. Look for healthier alternatives such as Zevia.

Coriander seeds. Steep seeds in water for about an hour. Strain & sip the infusion throughout the day.

Crackers. For lesser degrees of nausea, using any bland food as part of a remedy line-up should be considered, but it isn't something that works alone for severe cases. * *In HG circles, being offered crackers is a joke, even garnering its own term; "crackered." On a parched throat it may choke the dehydrated woman.*

Curry leaves. Extract juice from 15-20 leaves, mix with lime juice, add honey and drink 2-3 cups/day to tame stomach.

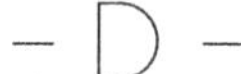

Dairy Products. Some doctors recommend dairy to soothe the queasy stomach and give added protein to the diet, while others say "no," because dairy is hard to digest. Certified raw milk from pasture fed cows from a trustworthy source is better utilized by the body. (Read, "The Raw Milk Revolution," by David Gumpert). Cheese can be tolerated better than milk, for some.

Distractions. Really! The morning sickness still remains, but the intensity can be briefly deferred. It doesn't always work. When it does, you'll have brief periods of rest. Some distraction include: talking on the phone, watching a movie, laughing, having someone visit with you, going somewhere, or doing something you enjoy and can get "lost" in.

Drugs / Medications. As the very last resort, of coarse. Seek counsel from your doctor. A helpful organization to go to with questions about the safety of any medication taken during pregnancy is motherrisk.org. If you go this route, you'll still need to maintain a remedy line-up so that the medication can be used as little as possible.

– E –

Eating. Small, frequent amounts would be the ideal goal. I know you might not feel like eating, or your body might strongly object. But, keeping something in your stomach, even in the tiniest amount, can prevent a downward spiral of nausea, where lack of eating results in more nausea which causes less eating, ...so eat! Eat the things you are craving. Don't force yourself to eat something that currently revolts you. Choose the best sounding items, even if it's not on the top of the health charts. Sweet, sour, salty, bland, crunchy, hard, soft, liquidy, sugary... If you're feeling guilty about bad food choices, know that you'll be able to make more consistently healthy decisions as the nausea lessens. Just do the best you can to eat well, and nourish your body.

It has been suggested that our body's requirements for food are paralleled by the baby's needs for nourishment. As the baby is rapidly developing so our need to continually replenish the baby's supply of food is required. This is achieved by our eating every few hours. Eat as healthy as you possibly can, as often as you can. But, if it doesn't quite work out the ideal way during your day, the baby will take what it needs from you, even depleting your reserves. Get back to the healthy eating track, when you can.

And when eating - go slow. Take little bites; let it absorb slowly into your system. No matter how hungry or thirsty you are, always eat & drink sloooow.

Entrox. (Contains Perilla seed) This combo helps detoxify the liver and aid in digestion. It is recommended to be taken pre- pregnancy along with milk thistle (280 mg) along with a product called Absorb Aid 3X a day.

Enzymes. Digestive enzymes taken before every meal can significantly help your taxed and slowed digestive system to help alleviate nausea.

Essential Oils. During pregnancy, your sense of smell is heightened. Pleasant aromas such as oil of Peppermint, Spearmint, Lemon, Lavender, Ginger, Sandalwood or Chamomile can alleviate nausea for some. The safest essential oils to use on your skin during pregnancy are those from flowers.

Mix with coconut oil and massage into skin. 3 drops to 1 tablespoon carrier oil. Take a warm bath with 6-8 drops of the essential oil. Don't apply undiluted essential oils to your skin or take them internally. Make sure the oils are pure and certified. Inhale either directly from the bottle or pour up to 4 drops of one of the essential oils on a tissue and breathe in. Repeat as needed.

These are the essential oils to avoid during pregnancy: bay leaves, clove, basil, clary sage, marjoram, oregano, thyme and wintergreen.

Exercise. Some moms have greatly benefited from continuing their exercise regime. If you can do it, that would be great! Overall, our body functions so much better when it is exercised! Make sure to stop when you feel weak or dizzy. If you can't talk through the routine, your baby isn't getting enough oxygen, either. Make sure to not start something fast paced, if you haven't already built up to that level.

– F –

Fennel Seeds. Has a licorice taste. Chinese folk medicine remedy. Make fennel tea, add honey & lemon and sip slowly to aid queasiness. It is found in a lot of combo prenatal herbal remedies and vitamins. Or, chew seeds.

Fermented Foods. Many nutrients and enzymes. Loads of help with digestion. Some yummy probiotic drinks are Kombucha and Kefir. Kimchi.

Fresh Air / Altitude. In summer, a fan with aromatherapy directly in my face would ease my nausea, in winter, continual fresh air from open windows or doors would help. A change of scenery, location, and surroundings, can be helpful. If you live in a noisy, smelly place see if you can take short vacation trips, or stay with someone who lives in a more peaceful environment. Go somewhere that you can find quiet rest with fresh air. ****A special note about summer.*** Heat can intensify nausea. (And in winter if you have the heater set too high, it can make the air stale and contribute to nausea, too). Stay in places where you can get a steady supply of fresh, cool air.

Frozen ...anything! If there is a food you like - freeze it! Do this before you need it. Peeled, cut, and frozen grapes can help. If anyone offers to do this for you….let them! Invest in a portable refrigerator/freezer, or use an ice chest to have by your bed so that you can get this food with minimal effort during the night or early morning. Sometimes the effort in retrieving the food is not worth it when you are already feeling nauseous. ***Great foods to freeze:*** Watermelon, Cherries-pitted, Honeydew, Cantaloupe.

– G –

Ginger. A very popular recommendation. A rule of thumb is to take it until you can burp it. Try anything and everything ginger: fresh leaves, roots, capsules, teas, and blended tinctures, grated, pickled, candy, gum, juice, ginger cookies, crackers, and ginger ale. Many studies conclude the positive impact ginger has on nausea relief. For the powdered capsules: Taking 250 mg 4/day is the general recommendation.

- Or ½ teaspoon of the powder every 4 hours (make tea).
- Or ¼ oz. of the fresh root to chew on.

One source says to take up to 25 capsules per day for complete control of severe nausea and vomiting throughout the pregnancy.

Precautions: it is not recommended to take over 1,000 mg of ginger per day, and also there is a warning about not taking for more than 4 days in a row. Since nausea usually lasts more than 4 days, it would be a safeguard to use ginger along with another remedy. Rotating it in and out, as it works best for you.

Gum. Peppermint flavor is good. I absorbed as much of the pepperminty flavor I could get out of a stick, and then went for another one. I went through several packs a day. This has helped several other women as well. If you can only stand chewing for a few seconds, then spit it out and try again later. It is worth it to use and discard as you are able. My highest recommendation for gum: PEELU. A natural gum that can be found at Health Food Stores. It has Xylitol in it which dually helps prevent tooth decay and is a natural sweetener.

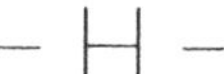

Herbs. Use them in teas, tinctures, capsules, candies, fresh, etc from high quality, trusted sources. Make sure to discuss with your health care provider. These are all the most recognized herbs which are considered safe & effective for morning sickness:

- Milk Thistle
- Ginger
- Peppermint
- Red Raspberry Leaf
- Slippery Elm Bark
- Oats & Oat Straw
- Lemon Balm
- Perilla seed

Home Health Care /Hospital (IV Fluids). For HG Moms. A lot of insurance plans will cover this. Ask your OB or midwife to write a prescription for it. I highly recommend! *This was a lifesaver for me. Not only did I NOT need to be in hospital surroundings. I could look forward to the days* *my nurse would come and visit. The home health nurses showed a lot of sympathy . The helpful visits broke up the monotony of the days. My fluids were continuous through the IV, vitamins were added in and this helped stop the downward cycle of throwing up at regular intervals.*

Homeopathy. Combinations can sometimes be more effective than singularly. Homeopaths suggest starting with remedies labeled 6c. Take these every two to eight hours, as needed. I've also seen suggestions for every 15 minutes until relief. The frequency of dosage varies with the condition and the individual. Sometimes a dose may be required several times an hour; other times a dose may be indicated several times a day; and in some situations, one dose per day (or less) can be sufficient. If no response is seen within a reasonable amount of time, select a different remedy. Top six homeopathic remedies for nausea: **Arsenicum Album, Carbo Vegetalis, Ignatia, Ipecacuanha, and Nux Vomica.**

A homeopath can put together a personal combination for you. Here is a link to find a homeopath near you: http://www.hpathy.com *Caution: If you are going to see a practitioner, ask questions and be aware of their beliefs.*

Remember: Do not consume any strong mint flavor 15 minutes before or after taking any homeopathic remedy. And do not take other food or drink within the same 15 minute period.

Interesting Note - A homeopathic formula marketed to dogs & cats to treat nausea from motion sickness. It contains the following 100% herbal and homeopathic ingredients: Zingiber officinalis (ginger). Mentha piperita (Mint) Kalium phosphate (Kali. phos.). Aconite C30, Cocculus C30, Pulsatilla vulgaris C6, and Lactose (inactive ingredient). You sprinkle this all natural formula on your tongue (that IS a valuable way to get something down). These ingredients are the same remedies people use! And it's in one combination. Pet owner testimonials: http://www.nativeremedies.com/petalive/easytravel-canine-travel-sickness-remedy.html - If someone tries this - I'd like to know.

Honey. Honey can give you a natural sugar boost, and provide you with some nutrients. Find raw, unfiltered honey for maximum nutrients.

— | —

Ice. This is a wonderful strategy for helping to relieve morning sickness. While water is hard to keep down, ice, if crushed, and taken in small amounts can sit in your mouth and melt. As it slowly gets absorbed, it is much easier to keep down, and the coolness of it can help nausea, too!

Instructions for Red Raspberry Leaf Tea Slushy:

Red Raspberry Leaf tea, long purported to bring balance to female hormones, especially during pregnancy. Putting RRL tea in blender with ice is good, but can be too watery. Here's another way to have it:

1- If you have an ice tea maker, put ½ cup of bulk fresh red raspberry leaves into filter. Use suggested amount of water, omitting the ice. Otherwise, try a big pot of water on the stove and toss 5-6 tea bags in after water is boiling.

2- When it cools, pour into 3 or 4 ice cube trays and freeze (the smaller the cubes, the easier it is to blend and get the best consistency for eating).

3- When frozen, store ice cubes into a gallon Ziploc bag, and start over if you want to stockpile.

4- When ready, take about 10-12 ice cubes and put into a good blender or ice crusher...get the ice to look like snow.

If someone else can do this whole process for you...even better! Use a spoon to take small amounts at a time (a plastic spoon may feel better in your mouth than metal...especially if you already have that metallic taste).

Remember, whatever you decide to freeze, crush it to have the smallest consistency you can. Smaller is better.

Ice Cream. Rice Cream, Almond Milk, any frozen desert can help. This is one food that produced significant results for many. Choose organic and/or a brand that has no preservatives, additives, etc.

Information. One of the most important things you can do is learn about nausea. That can be half the battle. Once a nauseous mom knows how to deal with it she can turn her attention to be more productive in finding ways to relieve it. See the Resource section to find links for other morning sickness info and to connect with other women who have or are experiencing it.

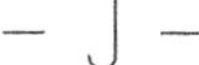

Japanese Miso Soup. This did wonders for some.

Jell-O. Any flavor. Eat it very slowly. Slurp it! Have someone make it from grass fed gelatin sources to avoid artificial ingredients.

– K –

K and C combination. In one study, women who took 5 mg of vitamin K and 25 mg of vitamin C per day reported the complete disappearance of morning sickness within three days. Most nutritionally oriented doctors use higher amounts of vitamin C (500–1,000 mg). These vitamins, it is said, are to be used in conjunction with each other via medical injection. Find a healthcare provider who can do this.

Kinesiology. Muscle testing. This is when the patient holds a substance the body may be allergic to or helped by. The doctor monitors how strong or weak the body's response is to it. Independent studies have been inconclusive as to the validity of such treatments.

Caution: Discernment is needed before participating in these therapies. Some principles can be scientifically proven and are reasonable to understand. Yet, they are mixed in with sketchy psychological and spiritual nuances. ***My advice:*** *When in doubt, do without.*

– L –

Lemon. .... Wedges, in water, aromatherapy. ***Everything lemon.*** Sip it, suck on it, smell it...Put the tincture lemongrass drops onto a washcloth. Keep it near you at all times. Inhale deeply and then breathe out slow. Keep the cloth in a Ziploc bag for easy portability. I know sucking on lemons can be hard on tooth enamel, but if you are in a survival mode that doesn't really matter to you. It helps the nausea. You can rinse out mouth well after each use.

Lemon Balm. The herb. Make an infusion with the dried herb or use 2 tsp. of fresh herb per cup of water. Drink up to 5 cups a day. Crush the fresh leaf between your fingers and rub onto your skin. Add the daily dose to a bath.

Lifesavers/Altoids. Peppermint Lifesavers or Altoids can help. Always a basic help for me in all my pregnancies.

Lights. Keep them dim. Avoid flashing and bright lights!

Lollipops. They can help. You don't need a special 'nausea" brand. Buy organic!

Loose-fitting clothes. This is something that might be obvious, but if you have anything causing even slight pressure around your abdomen, it could be increasing your nausea.

– M –

Magnesium. 500-750mg. Due to excess cortisol in our system during pregnancy, our blood sugar goes through huge spikes and crashes. This results in fatigue and nausea. Normally, magnesium balances cortisol levels but our pregnancy hormones can inhibit the ability to absorb magnesium leading to a cycle where the excess stress hormones cause nausea, which causes stress, etc. Take as a capsule or powder along with calcium for max absorption. Or try magnesium oil. A reputable brand is Ancient Minerals. Another way to absorb magnesium is to take a 30 minute bath in Epsom salts. (1/2 - 1 cup).

Magnetic Therapy. Sea bands. A lot of moms say this works for them. My mom made her own nausea remedy by using magnets bought from her local store. She used masking tape to hold them unto pressure points on her wrist and she said it helped her immensely. It was much cheaper than buying the manufactured version. A homemade version may work for you, too.

Milk Thistle. (Standardized to contain at least 70% silymarin) I have had many positive testimonials on the benefits of milk thistle. The form (for absorbability) and frequency of this supplement could affect the outcome. The liquid form would be best (www.trilightherbs.com). And start as soon as you can before conceiving. Milk thistle has been recommended to be taken along with AbsorbAid. (Amazon.com)

Molasses. This has iron and vitamin B in it!! If your throat is raw from vomiting stomach acids, or you have acid reflux, molasses helps coat your throat while providing nutrition.

Morning Sickness Magic. It has a lot of great ingredients in it. Helps some moms.

Morning Sickness Balm. I have heard many times over about it's success. (www.mountainmeadowherbs.com)

Morning Well CD. It takes about 40 minutes. *MorningWell* recommends you stop once you feel better. I listened to it at various times, for varying number of minutes according to how I felt. I played it for about 2 1/2 weeks. It was played it at a level that I could hear conversations going on around me. These are the pros/cons that I found:

PROS- No hypnosis, no drugs, no subliminal messages.

CONS: It didn't always work. After a while, the music annoyed me.

Did it work? Maybe.....sometimes. This is the link for the studies which showed it helped others: http://www.morningwell.co.uk/nhsstudy.htm

Movement/Motions.

- Moving exaggeratedly slow can really help reduce nausea.
- Beds cause too much movement, sleep on the floor or couch.
- Being a passenger in the car can be hard. Sit up front. Even better, be in the driver's seat. Chew gum.
- Rocking yourself slowly in a rocking chair or on the floor.
- When you first wake up, **before your first movement.** eat something little.

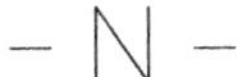

Nuts. Cashews, hazelnuts, almonds, walnuts, pecans,... High in protein, they are small and easy to carry with you. Snack on throughout day. Try nut butters, too.

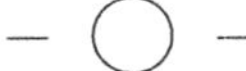

Olives. According to the National Library of Medicine, there are a number of symptoms that present themselves as a result of motion sickness, including increased salivation, which is the body's way of protecting the teeth from the high doses of acid accompanied by vomit. Olives contain tannins that, when released in the mouth, work to dry saliva-first eliminating the symptom and then the body's instinct to follow suit. The treatment is only effective during the early stages of nausea, when the salivation changes first appear. Choose organic. Find close to natural products with no artificial colors or preservatives.

Omega 3's. Certain types of fish are especially good. Mackerel, tuna, and mullet are some. These are high in Omega 3 fatty acids which are thought to also help reduce the risk of high blood pressure during pregnancy. Fish also has B6. Stay away from the clams, oysters and shrimp. A good source for the best digestible form is fermented cod liver oil. I highly recommend Greenpastures.com fermented cod liver oil mixed with butter fat. (By the way, it also cured my son's asthma)!

Oranges. Citrus fruits are all beneficial. Peel, section & freeze. Suck on one at a time. Orange sherbet. Orange flavored tea. Icey!

– P –

Papaya. Fresh, juice, dehydrated...in all forms it's supposed to calm a nauseous stomach. Another food you can chop and freeze!

Peach Tree Leaf. A study was done that says it helps nausea. I notice this ingredient is found in some combo remedies.

Peppermint. Candy, gum, fresh mint leaves, tea, aromatherapy. This helps! Especially the gum. PEELU gum has xylitol which is better for your health and teeth than sugar substitutes found in most gum.

Pickles. Dill or sweet. Dill is supposed to calm the stomach. Sweet, to satisfy the sweet & sour craving.

Popsicles. In any season! Make these from everything. Tea, Juice, mashed fruit, sherbet, yogurt, kefir,...etc.

Prayer. Never underestimate the power of healing from God, if it is His will. Through prayer in Jesus name, He can give you the strength, resources and endurance to overcome any trials. (Good ministry: rzim.org/)

Preggie Pops or B-Natal TheraPops. Regular organic candy in flavors you like, will work just as well.

Pregnancy Tea. Special nutrients for pregnant moms. Make it into an ice slushy. If you decide to drink it hot, then sip it very slowly.

Probiotics. A changing digestive system due to fluctuating hormones cause the hormone surges at different times and can create indigestion problems causing yeast infections and bloating. Having lots of good bacteria in your system can benefit you. How to get it there: 1) Buy acidophilus capsules and sprinkle them on anything you eat. 2) Drink very small sips of flavored kefir. Kefir is supposed to be more digestible than yogurt.
3) Fermented foods & drinks. Sip Kombucha. Try Beet kvass, ginger ale, or sauerkraut. They all have beneficial bacteria and may help reduce intestinal upsets. There are many fun varieties of different kinds and flavors in the stores.

Pro-G-Yam cream. Progesterone cream. Suggested application 2x - morning and bedtime. As always, before using hormones, talk it over with a knowledgeable health care professional.

Protein. "Eat high protein snacks to prevent low blood sugar resulting in less nausea" theory.

Sometimes, I would eat every two hours throughout the day, and continue that schedule in the night, to keep the right foods in my system to keep my blood sugar level up. Cottage cheese, tuna, milk, peanut butter, almonds....any high protein food will help. Include protein in your small frequent meal plan.

– Q –

Quiet! Noises, and in particular loud or monotonous noises, can worsen nausea. Try to minimize all sounds that could exasperate your already unstable nausea. Listen to calm and soothing music, or sounds.

– R –

Red Raspberry Leaf. Making this herb into an ice slushy was my favorite relief. Taking it in the liquid tincture form can be a quick and easy way to get it in your system, also. I've used it with every one of my pregnancies.

Rest. Slowing down and taking naps can lessen the stress your body is going through. Wear dark glasses and get comfortable, using lots of pillows. Put soothing music on and breathe deeply. Relax and enjoy this season.

– S –

Sancuso. An anti-nausea drug patch. Most doctors have not heard of it yet. This patch lasts 5 days and is predicted to be the next big thing for HG moms. Smaller pharmacies can order fit for you, if big chains don't carry it. Pros: No constant medication reminders, reduces nausea. Cons: Expensive. At the time of this writing \$332.18 for one patch.

Salty Foods. You may just want to suck the salt off the food instead of actually eating the food. The Salt and Vinegar flavor potato chip can help dry up excess saliva, which can trigger nausea. Make sure your chips don't contain the fat substitute Olestra which can rob your body of important nutrients. Celtic Sea salt is best!

Salt Pack. For a soothing stomach remedy for vomit spasms: Take an old pillowcase, dampen it, fill it with 1 – 2 cups of warmed sea salt. Then let it cover your whole stomach area. This may be calming as it absorbs into your skin.

Sauerkraut. Any fermented food, really. Probiotic, minerals, vitamins.

Seaweed. For magnesium.

Showers. Take them often! Being clean, smelling clean, and ridding yourself of the toxins that accumulate on your skin help decrease nausea. If you feel weak, put a chair in there.

Slippery Elm. The mucilage in slippery elm will soothe your stomach and intestines. 200 mg. 3x/day before meals. or chew 3-4 tablets before eating. Or try this: Make a broth out of barley and whole oats. Strain the grains and add slippery elm. You will probably have to mix in a blender to blend well. Add miso, tamari, or other pleasing seasonings.

Snacks or small, frequent meals. It is better to eat a little bit of food more often than larger amounts a few times a day.

Soaked grains. Steel cut oats and other grains, if soaked overnight with ACV, whey or lemon juice, and allowed to cook slowly on low heat will be more easily digestible and soothe an upset stomach.

Spirulina. Micronutrients. Essential for maximum nutrition support. Mix in smoothies or sprinkle on food.

Support. Know that you are not battling nausea alone! Join a forum. (See Resource section) Stay in touch with sympathetic friends, read books from survivors. Keep in contact with a caring health care provider. Accept help from those who care about you. Surround yourself with thoughtful people who focus on the positive. Read the Bible. Pray.

Stress. Eliminate it. This can throw nausea into a higher level. It will exasperate your already delicate system. Remember: ***Rest helps stress.***

Spa. Get pampered. You deserve it! (Just be aware of strong smells that may be there such as perms & nails). Getting the spa treatment, like a relaxing massage, can help you rest and feel rejuvenated.

– T –

Tea. Herbal tea. Can taste better than water, for some. Contains nutrients. Many varieties. Stay away from caffeine. Some blends below:

Morning Sickness Tea Blend #1:
Lemongrass,
chamomile, nettle,
with a subtle hint of ginger.

Morning Sickness Tea Blend #2:
Peppermint,
spearmint, nettle,
red raspberry leaf.

Teeth. Dental floss and toothbrushes can exasperate your gag reflex.

To brush your teeth without gagging: Use your finger with some toothpaste on it or a n infant toothbrush designed for toddlers (www.rightstart.com) to brush your teeth. Without the long handle of regular brushes, this can help you continue good oral hygiene.

Use toothpaste without fluoride. Tom's of Maine and Spry offer a fluoride-free alternative. *Note: When you can't brush because of nausea, at least rinse out with a natural mouthwash. (Tom's of Maine, food grade hydrogen peroxide, colloidal silver, ..) Try briefly oil pulling, when it seems possible, with a very small amount of coconut or sesame oil.*

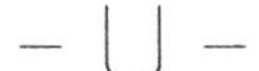

Unisom/Vitamin B6 Combo. Vitamin B6 supplements can reduce symptoms of mild to moderate nausea, but do not usually help with vomiting. The non-prescription sleep-aid, Unisom, contains Doxylamine, that studies have shown is effective in reducing nausea. When combined with vitamin B6, this duo seems to have great results. Combinations formulations that are time released are available for the initial treatment of nausea as Diclectin in Canada and Diclegis in the United States. As always, consult with your doctor first before taking any medication. Contact www.motherrisk.com for more info on drugs in pregnancy.

– V –

Vegetable Broth. Soothing and nutritious. Make a big batch and freeze in smaller containers for a quick meal supplement.

Vegetable Juice. Juice lots of celery, carrots, spinach and an apple, with a slice of ginger to allay nausea and get max nutrition! Sip slooooowly. Freeze some for later.

Vitamins. Try liquid vitamins for faster, easier absorption. Children's vitamins can be more tolerable. The iron in your prenatal vitamins could be increasing your nausea. Ask for a non-iron vitamin to be prescribed. (The herb Nettle contains natural iron in it. As does liquid chlorophyll).

What to do when those prenatal vitaminas are just way too big to swallow, keep down, or cause stomach upset:

- Liquid whole food supplements. Vitacost.com has good options for liquid prenatal multivitamins.
- Grind up solid vitamins then sprinkle on food or blend in smoothies.
- Take children's chewable vitamins (smaller & pleasant tasting).
- Fruits and vegetables in any shape and form you can get them. (***See JuicePlus.com)***
- Use your own juicer to drink kale, carrot, apple juice. ***Find many veg/fruit drink choices at your local health food store.***

– W –

Wasabi. Spicy flavor from root that has helped some moms with nausea. For those who simply cannot afford the genuine root, most cooks say the wasabi powder will work nearly as well as the wasabia japonica.

Water. If you can pinch your skin and it doesn't bounce back, or if you touch your tongue and it is dry, then you are dehydrated. It can be difficult to drink when you have nausea. Use a straw. Suck on ice. Take very slow, very small amounts. Do not drink with meals (wait 30 min. to 1 hour). Never gulp. As often as you can, drink (sip) water. (Read, "Your Body's Many Cries for Water," by F. Batmanghelidj).

I have a friend who bought a HUGE, mega jug from a convenience store. She fills it with water in the morning and sips it throughout the day. If you can toss in a lemon slice, cucumber, mint leaves, or add ACV even better. It is important to stay hydrated. Keep your doctor or midwife aware, if you are not drinking 6-8 glasses a day. Another friend has a water app on her phone to remind her when to drink water.

3 ways to get water into your system without drinking it:

1- Eat or drink or suck on fruits and vegetables that have a high water content. (iceberg lettuce, melons, grapes, ...).

2- Take a warm bath to absorb water through your skin. *Note: If you are feeling faint, make sure you have someone who can help assist you in doing this.*

3- In extreme situations, you can keep your mouth moist by biting down gently on a damp wash cloth.

Watermelon... is the perfect frozen fruit because it has a high water and sugar content, and replaces the electrolytes lost when throwing up. I've heard from many moms who have been helped by watermelon, that it was the one food that got them through the worst of times.

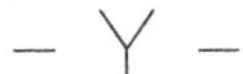

Yam, Wild. Use with caution. It is a tonic herb so it should be taken in small amounts over a period of several days. 1 to 2 tsp three times of day of the dried wild yam herb, or as a tincture take 2 to 4 ml three times daily. It balances hormones and nourishes the liver. Sip the tea to alleviate morning sickness.

Yogurt popsicles. They don't melt as fast as juice popsicles and have more nutrition. You could try making kefir pops, too.

– Z –

Zinc. Plasma zinc levels were lower in pregnant women with morning sickness. Zinc can balance blood sugar levels, stabilize metabolic rates, and strengthen the immune system. Current recommendations are 15mg. Some foods zinc can be found in are spinach, toasted wheat germ, beef & lamb.

Chapter 4

Strategies for Success

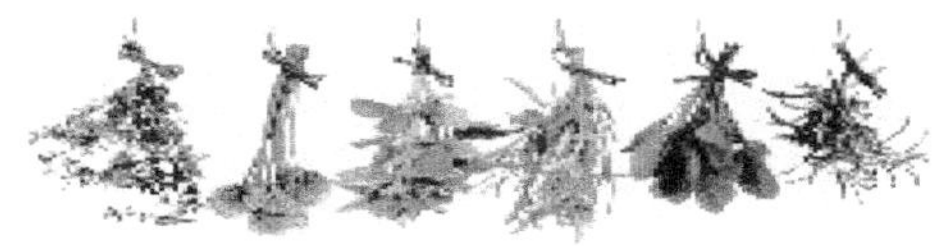

We gain strength, and courage, and confidence by each experience in which we really stop to look fear in the face... we must do that which we think we cannot.

-Eleanor Roosevelt

What's your plan? Use the next few pages to organize your strategies.

Your Personal Remedy Wrap-Up

People I Can Call When I Need an Encouraging Word:

____

____

Those I Can Email, Text or Chat with for Distractions:

____

____

Friends/Family Who Will Come Over and Help:

____

____

Places I Can Go to Experience Comfort:

____

____

Book/Movies that May Offer Me Solace:

____

____

Organizations that Can Assist Me:

____

Foods that I Feel Like Trying:

____

____

Beverages that I can Sip:

____

____

Salty Foods:

____

____

Sweet Foods:

____

____

Sour Foods:

____

____

Bland Foods:

____

____

Daily Goals

First thing in the morning:

Throughout the day:

Before Bed:

My Morning Sickness Journal

Date:	Time:	Trigger?	What I did.	Prevention.
5/12/12	3:30pm	nap	yogurt popsicle	eat before nap

Date:	Time:	Trigger?	What I did.	Prevention.

- Go to MyMorningSickness.com to download this E-Journal free.-

"Women know the way to rear up children [to be just].
They know a simple, merry, tender knack
of tying sashes, fitting baby shoes,
And stringing pretty words that make no sense,
And kissing full sense into empty words."

—Elizabeth Barrett Browning, poet

Chapter 5

Extreme Nausea

Hyperemesis Gravidarum Support

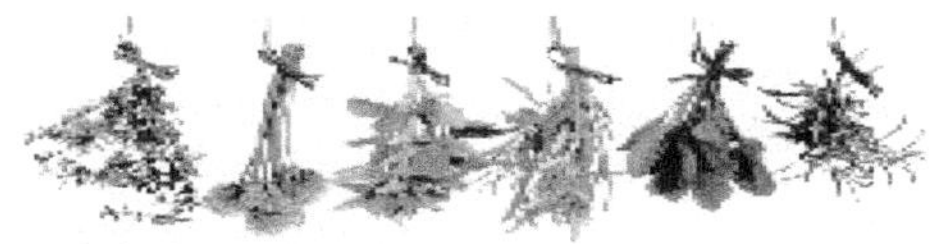

"A ship under sail and a big-bellied woman,
Are the handsomest two things that
can be seen common."

-Benjamin Franklin

Warning Signs of Severe NVP

*(Nausea and Vomiting in Pregnancy)

-You experience 4-6 hours of nothing staying down.

-You are not urinating, or it is a dark color when you do.

-You are losing weight.

-Your vomit contains blood or bile.

-You vomit more than 5 times a day.

-When you vomit is prolonged with dry heaving.

*If you recognize any of these symptoms find a doctor or midwife to monitor you!

"There is a comfort in the strength of love;
'Twill make a thing endurable, which else
Would overset the brain, or break the heart."

– William Wordsworth

My Story

My husband, and I, went to register our first home birth at the local county office. As we were filling out the forms, the friendly clerk inquired, "Did you have any complications?" I emphatically answered, "Oh yes! Morning sickness!" After politely smiling, she said, "That isn't considered a complication." *Really??* I remembered how I lived on the ground next to a throw up bowl for months because I couldn't physically move to the toilet due to exhaustion from dry heaving throughout the days and nights. I was so dehydrated that I was admitted to the hospital several times to have IV's of fluid, and multiple medications were prescribed. I lost weight - more than 15 lbs. in 2 months. The nausea was miserably torturing me. Hmm...not a complication.... well, I hoped it meant only few women suffered from it. I've learned a lot since then that I can share with you!

Your Story

On the next page are some powerful ways to look at your current situation. **Never lose a positive outlook.** Keep going. Pray. You can do it for your baby. Never give up! Don't think about tomorrow or next week, just get through this next minute. On the next page is a quiz I created when coming out of morning sickness from an earlier pregnancy. Can you relate?

If you aren't sure yet if you have severe nausea, you'll know after taking this quiz...

The Extreme Nausea Quiz

Motions

1. a) You feel queasy, sometimes.

   b) Your "morning" sickness never leaves.

2. a) Sudden, fast movements may make you feel queasy.

   b) Any movement, anytime, anywhere, has an impact on stomach contents coming back up.

3. a) Eating is an overall enjoyable experience that can help allay your nausea.

   b) If you can eat, you cautiously choose a food based on forethought about what might be the consequence of a trip back up.

4. a) When someone tells you to eat crackers and have small frequent meals, it is helpful.

   b) The advice lets you know that the person speaking does not understand what is going on with you.

5. a) Riding in cars and lying in bed are still functional things to do.

   b) These become your worst enemies because of the slightest non-initiated movement factor.

Daily Life

6. a) You are pretty much able to go about your day as usual in the same social circles.

   b) The floor, your bed, and the bathroom have become your new social circle.

7. a) You are concerned about possibly gaining weight.

   b) You are concerned about the weight you are losing.

8. a) All five of your senses may be heightened just a little.

   b) All five of your senses have grown to bionic proportions

9. a) The days go by rather quickly.

   b) The days go by so slowly and laboriously that you can count time by the milliseconds.

10. a) If you do throw up, it is fairly quick and it brings instant relief.

    b) Throwing up is a 10 minute heaving experience that brings momentarily relief before giving way to miserable, agonizing nausea once again.

Sleep

11. a) For the most part you are able to get a good night's sleep.

    b) Sleep is something you try to do in between bouts of nausea and throwing up.

12. a) 7-8 hours of sleep at night and maybe a nap during the day help you feel restful and energized.

    b) If a full night's sleep is obtained, and several naps taken during the day, you still feel like it has been a week since you closed your eyes.

Food

13. a) You may have certain food cravings and these bring satisfaction.

    b) Cravings are last hope efforts to relieve you of your queasy feeling, and must be satisfied within a very small window of time to prevent any further complications.

14. a) If something sounds good to eat, you fix it/find it and all is well.

    b) If something sounds good to eat, but you have to get it, then the odds of it staying down decrease proportionately with how much time/effort you gave.

15. a) You can drink water with no ill effect.

    b) Water has to be sipped, icy cold, held in your mouth for a predetermined amount of time, and slowly swallowed to keep it down.

Smells

16. a) Smells don't generally bother you, although you may avoiding certain scents.

    b) One brief whiff of something that doesn't even have a traceable odor to the average person can make you ill.

What Others are Saying

17. a) You have that pregnancy glow and others tell you so, even when you don't feel quite well.

    b) You're sick to your stomach most of the time, extremely miserable, and can't remember what if feels like to feel good.

18. a) People understand and sympathize with you.

    b) No one understands and can relate to you.

19. a) People generally sympathize with you about your queasiness problems and offer comfort.

    b) People don't know how to respond to your extreme sickness and offer words of "help" that often make you feel worse.

Summary

20. a) Labor will be more challenging than your nausea.

    b) Compared to "morning" sickness, you feel labor will be a breeze.

If you consistently chose answer 'b', you most likely have HG!!

HG Requires Extra Attention!

You can survive the emotional/physical downward spiral common with HG by ***faithfully remembering these 3 Things:***

1) **Stay in contact with your doctor/midwife.** Have a qualified health care professional monitor your health.

2) **Stay connected. Seek help from others.**

3) **Stay positive.** You are in a survivor mode. Hang on to a sense of humor and/or a hopeful disposition. This can help you not be utterly discouraged during this challenge.

Emotional Support in HG

If you are experiencing nausea so severe that you are finding it impossible to do the most simple and basic tasks, you most likely have Hyperemesis Gravidarum (HG). HG is the medical definition for the worst kind of morning sickness. A closer study of the Latin root words reveal the awful truth; hyper means "over"; emesis "vomiting"; and gravid arum, "pregnant state." Thus, excessive vomiting in pregnancy.

Excessive vomiting is considered vomiting more than 5 times a day. The medical definition doesn't fully describe the extent of this condition, though. I have my own personal definition: Severe, extreme, exhausting, persistent, constant, continuous, never-ending, life-changing nausea of pregnancy. Although a Latin word "Acer-extremus-adficio-pertinax-jugis-perpetuus-aeturnus-eturnus-mutatio gravidarum" would be a little hard to repeat when asked what is wrong! After preterm labor, hyperemesis is the second most common reason for hospital admission during the first half of a women's pregnancy.

When Others Don't Understand

Those closest to you may not be able to comprehend your misery. As you feel absolutely tortured on the inside, the presence of nausea can go completely unnoticed by them. When your head isn't in the toilet bowl, you may be told you look good and have a pregnancy glow! And, while these sincere compliments may be true, it can add further frustration that others do not understand how bad you are actually feeling.

I've included some resources in this chapter to share with your loved ones to give them ideas which enable them to better respond to your needs! Also, I've listed ways to help you keep your attitude up.

Applying the following suggestions are tools to help you achieve more success at staying on top of your pregnancy in thoughts, emotions, feelings and above life's current challenging nausea situations.

Rapid Responses

Most people don't know how to respond to an unfamiliar situation, so you may have heard a lot of "helpful" comments that weren't so helpful. I jotted down the most common and what I would have liked to hear, instead. :) Communicate with others about your needs. Let them know what you're thinking and keep a sense of humor when you hear...

1. "It's all in your head, just think positive."

   Better: "I know this is hard for you, can I help?"

2. "It couldn't be that bad, it's just morning sickness."

   (50,000 women are hospitalized every year).

   Better: "What a great job you are doing in nurturing this little one before it is born."

3. "I felt great during my pregnancy!"

   Better: "I'm sorry you aren't feeling well."

4. "I get it, but not as bad as you," or

   "I've never known anyone who gets as sick as you."

   Better: "I am here for you."

5. "Just eat crackers."

   Better: "What can I get for you right now?"

6. "Let me know if you need anything."

   Better: Be specific. "I would like to_________; would you be comfortable with that?"

7. "Have you tried...." (Yes, I did...*lots of times!!!!*)

   Better: "I bought_____for you. Do you want to try again?"

For Friends & Family of the Nauseous Mom:

1. Help with the duties and responsibilities that she is unable to do.
   Offer to do specific jobs that would help her, or her family.

2. Give her a card of encouragement.
   A small token of kindness can go a long way to encourage her.

3. If talking with someone is a good distraction for her, call or visit her.
   The days and nights go by very slowly depending on how sick she feels.

4. Send flowers or something pretty to look at. Beautiful things can be uplifting to see. Especially if she is grounded to one part of the house for most of the day.

5. Read to her. Write her a poem. Sing, if she wants you to. It's nice for her to know that she is remembered, as she feels the world going on without her.

6. Little gifts are always welcome. Any small thoughtful gesture can make a big difference for her spirit.

7. Use encouraging words and tender comments. This can be an emotionally trying experience and all conversations need to be optimistic and focus on the positive.

8. Humor can be a welcome addition to her day.
   A funny book, movie, or you ? Can you make her smile?
   Making her laugh can be a great relief.

9. Be willing to serve her. Change sheets, offer food, clean, etc...

10. Pray with her! 

What God Hath Promised!

God hath not promised
 Skies always blue,
Flower-strewn pathways
 All our lives through;
God hath not promised
 Sun without rain
Joy without sorrow,
 Peace without pain.

But God hath promised
 Strength for the day,
Rest for the labor,
 Light for the way,
Grace for the trials,
 Help from above,
Unfailing sympathy,
 Undying love.

– Annie Johnson Flint

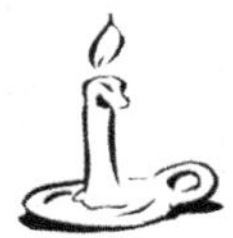

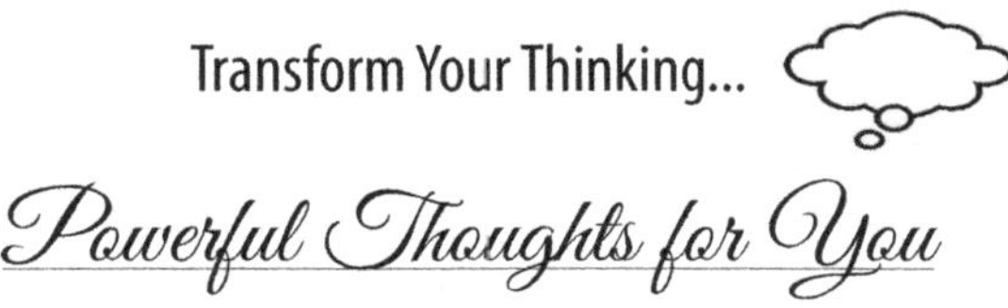

Transform Your Thinking... Powerful Thoughts for You

Old Thought: How can I continue in this misery one more minute?

New Thought: I can take one minute at a time! Each minute I go through, brings me one more minute closer to my baby's birth.

Old Thought: I feel desperate, disappointed and frustrated about the nausea being so intense.

New Thought: Small steps are big successes. I won't give up on continuing to experiment with different ways to achieve relief.

Old Thought: No one can truly understand this constant agony.

New Thought: There is a whole world of women feeling just like me who made it through. I can find one sympathetic friend. (Look in the blog section).

Old Thought: I don't remember what it feels like to feel good.

New Thought: I'm a survivor! I can focus on how far I've come and look ahead with hope. Nausea doesn't last forever.

> "When you feel like giving up,
> remember why you held on for so long in the first place."

Your Thoughts...

"Only a life lived for others is worth living."

-Albert Einstein

Post a List for Others to Know Your Needs:

Thank you for helping me...

Prepare a Meal That I Can Eat Right Now

Cook & Freeze Mea's for Later

Clean the Refrigerator

Vacuum

Dust/Spider webs

Run Laundry

Empty Trash

Go to the Store for Me

Plan an Activity for My Children

Clean Bathrooms

Just Visit with Me

Run Errands

....

....

Special Considerations:

I'm sensitive to noise.

No synthetic air fresheners, please.

No cologne or scented candles.

....

Thank you so much!!

"When you get to the end of your rope,
tie a knot and hang on."

–Franklin D. Roosevelt

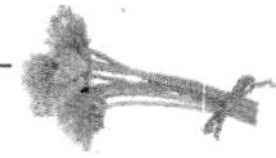

HAVE YOU EVER FELT LIKE THIS?

"The nausea was horrible."

"I don't know if I can do this again!"

The next few pages are letters from pregnant Moms who wrote me in the midst of their severe nausea. Their sincere and thoughtful letters show the reality of their struggles. These women love their family and unborn baby, and at the same time are experiencing fear, disappointment, frustration, and confusion.

Often we can find comfort knowing others have been on the path where we now trod. They made it through, and you can too. You are not alone! Maybe you can empathize with some of their feelings.

"Hello Wendy, thank you so much for your email. As soon as I woke up and went into the kitchen, the smell made me throw up. (well, I guess there was nothing to throw up, just wretching) To see your response this morning, made me feel better :)
I am really struggling with fear of what is to come. With my last pregnancy, I was bed bound with an IV line and a home health nurse visiting every couple of days. Even with zofran, i still had the debilitating nausea. I couldn't even the stand the smell of my children. :(My mother-in-law came to help, b/c I could not care for the kids and I think even my husband went into depression, with his life partner completely out of it!!!! The thought of what is coming makes me cry even as I type out this email. Thank you for taking the time to read my email and thank you for spending your time and effort to help women with this! It's nice to read something other than "eat saltines". Sincerely, "K.C."

♡

Wendy - I just ordered your book and read the entire thing - I can't thank you enough for your hard work and love for the Lord. Let me tell you about me, I am now 4-5 weeks into my 12th pregnancy - all HG pregnancies. I have 5 live children - the rest lost to miscarriage (8-16 weeks gestation). I too home school. My HG is of the very severe type, sounds like maybe you can relate - torn bleeding throat, hospitalizations, completely bedridden, etc, etc. I just found out about 1-2 weeks ago that I am expecting - and I am pulling together a plan for myself. I am taking many supplements - and will try to make that ice mash you talked about!.... "C.B."

♡

"I just found your web site the other day and think it is fantastic that you have put together all this information about morning sickness. I have 7 children myself and have had the HG type with all of them!! I thought I was the only one out there who got it so bad yet still went on to have a decent sized family!! The worst thing about it was that no one quite knew what to do with me. I was surrounded by my mother-in-law and sisters-in-law and female friends who never even got a hint of sickness with their pregnancies. I remember one sister-in-law who was trying to help me feel better told me that in some of her pregnancies water tasted a bit funny sometimes!! So all think that there must be something deeply wrong with me or it is all in my head!!..." - "G.L."

"... I'm 20 and I just had my first baby on October 10th. I had a really bad experience with Hyperemesis gravidarum. I lived on my couch and I was in so much pain. My body ached worse than the flu and I couldn't stand for a few seconds without passing out. I threw up at least every 30 minutes without eating or the minute I tried eating. The hospital and OB I went to didn't take me seriously. Neither did my family. They all told me that every pregnant woman goes through it and to just eat crackers and it'll calm the nausea. I desperately needed an IV and the hospital made we wait 7 hours for it. They gave me nausea medicine through an IV which later they told me wasn't safe for pregnancy. They gave me Zofran to take home and said it would dissolve or to chew it. After I took it the pharmacist told me it wasn't to chew or dissolve and doing that will overdose. I got the right Zofran and it did nothing for nausea. Once I started to recover and could keep food down I was still losing weight from my body eating my muscle and fat thinking I'm still starving. I felt everyone was very insensitive to me and the only person I had to care for me was my husband who was laid off from his job a few months before all of this. We moved and now he has a job and we have a beautiful baby boy named Kevin (It means "Handsome" and I knew he was going to be BEAUTIFUL). he's always been happy and healthy inside of me despite how sick I was. Now he's a sweet, well behaved and perfectly healthy baby. I had told everyone after I had him that he'd have to be an only child and then I felt God telling me I needed to trust in him and allow him to decide how many children he wants us to have. My husband agreed and I feel peace knowing God is in control. However, I can't help but worry about going through that again with nobody and having to take care of my baby when I can't even care for myself." - "L.R."

"...I have 12 days left of this [nausea] before my scheduled C-section on July 14th. I'm currently confined to bed for about 22 hours per day. I can't drive anymore. I can't take care of my children at all (thank God I'm married to a teacher home on Summer vacation!). My days are spent like the women in the article. This is not a "poor me" statement or a request for sympathy"..."Yes, this is our last baby. I was told that I won't survive another pregnancy. My doctor said, "Your three boys need their momma more than you need a fourth child. Back to bed now." Love "V.L."

"..... I have had Hyperemasis with all my Children, I am on number 6 and it is horrible. I am usually the positive cheerful about life in my home and I am discouraged this time around. I prayed that God would heal me of this tourment each time and my heart is a little broken. I know that Gods Plans are higher and that he has a purpose through all of this. Every thing from smell, reading, light noise act makes me sick. It is over the top. I am a home school mom , with a 12, 9, 7,5, and 19 month old. I have been on IV for a month and hospitalized twice. Once for my kidneys having issues from hydration and the other my esophagus swelling from the acid of vomiting. I throw up ALL day and even puke my way out of sleeping. My faith is usually strong and up until this point we have been a family that has left God in charge of our womb□ I am terrified to have to do this again. The statement it self sounds horrible, and I am ashamed to say is how I feel right now. I ADORE my Children and I am so very blessed by them. My body is really having issues with these severe pregnancies. This one is really hard. I have done the hospital thing many times, the Iv many times□ but now I get NO relief. My husband has hired a nanny for the next few weeks to see if a rest will help me. I feel bad about that but the Doctors are not SEEING any progress□ I may have to be on nutrition bags soon. Please pray for me. I CAN USUALLY HANDLE ALOT BUT THIS ONE IS HAS BEEN THE HARDEST. I am trying to encourage my self each day so that my poor little baby does not feel a sick , and discouraged mama. Thank you for your prayers." -S.E.

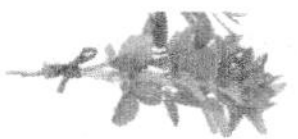

The following personal counsel was originally written for Moms who were considering future pregnancies after coming through a very challenging nausea experience.

These are practical principles that will also be helpful to those Moms who are currently struggling with overcoming nausea at this very moment.

> "Nothing in life is to be feared.
> It is only to be understood."
>
> – Marie Curie

From One Queasy Mother to Another

Nausea is hard! It can be an absolute life-changer when it hits hard, affecting everything we do. And, everyone in our life is somehow impacted by our circumstance, as well. I'll share with you what God has taught my husband and I when we have faced our challenging situations. As a Christian, I offer these thoughts from a distinctly biblical perspective.

Why does HG happen to ME? Why do I get hit harder with nausea than others? The reasons are numerous: exposure to toxins, genetics, lifestyle habits, etc.. We live in a fallen world (Genesis 3). Consequently, by the very fact we live on earth we will have to endure trials and hardships. A great blessing as a Christian is knowing our sovereign God allows us to go through trials ultimately for our benefit (Rom. 8:28). As our faith is tested, we are being conformed to the image of Christ, and He will produce good fruit in us through difficulties. In all of life's trials, we need to trust Him with the circumstances and outcome, faithfully submitting to whatever task is at hand. So, personally, if trials need to occur anyway, then I'll glory that a small part of my shaping can occur while I am growing and nurturing a new child!

How do you know God's will for you? When not sure about what God's will is, our situation can overwhelm us due to doubts. "Was this right? How could I do this to myself? What about my family?" God wants to guide you. Pray and read His Word. He understands where we are at, and where he wants to take us. We have an utter dependence on Him for our daily direction. That is why it is essential to be in His word constantly, in prayer unceasingly, and in fellowship with His people continually. We know He will walk us through challenges when we are faithful in following him.

Preparation and Application. My husband and I are always in prayer about all aspects of our family. Once pregnancy is confirmed, I prepare for a four-pronged approach: spiritual, emotional, physical and mental. Below are the things I do to guard against challenging situations from becoming debilitating ones:

Spiritually: 1) Make sure my will is submitted to His will. 2) Memorize and meditate on Scripture. 3) Solicit the help of Christian sisters who will pray, support and minister to me when needed. 4) Pray. 5) Listen to sermons.

Emotionally: 1) Stay positive. 2) Let myself cry when I need to. 3) But, keep my attitude in check. If I perceive I am becoming bitter, angry or depressed, I increase my time with the Lord. 4) Share my challenges with godly, optimistic people who will encourage me.

Mentally: 1) Focus on the positives. 2) Memorize key Scriptures dealing with where I am struggling. 4) Read edifying books. 5) Listen to uplifting music and/or Scripture. 6) Listen, watch and read funny things. 7) Choose a project that I can enjoy and become engrossed in when I'm in need of a good distraction.

Physically: 1) Eat healthy (include supplements, too) and exercise. 2) Prepare food to go in the freezer in advance. Make a menu and shop for food that anyone in the house can fix. 3) Have ready each remedy that can help to ease the nausea intensity. 4) Put an ice chest by my bed with food/drink. 5) Have a "things to do" box for the kids when I need extra time in bed. 6) Give my family pre-game instructions for what the next month(s) may entail. 7) As awful as I feel, get up, shower and dress nice daily. Looking sloppy will only increase my feelings of feeling icky! 8) Keep hydrated. 9) Stay on top of how I am feeling. Make sure to not fall into a downward cycle.

I have learned how to ease the morning sickness season by being prepared and relying on God. He gives wisdom, knowledge and understanding for what to do. and how to do it. He is sufficient to walk you through.

Comforting Scripture

"Peace I leave with you; my peace I give you. I do not give to you as the world gives. Do not let your hearts be troubled and do not be afraid." (John 14:27)

"Do not worry about anything, but in everything by prayer and supplication with thanksgiving let your requests be made known to God. And the peace of God, which surpasses all understanding, will guard your hearts and your minds in Christ Jesus. Finally, beloved, whatever is true, whatever is honorable, whatever is pleasing, whatever is commendable, if there is any excellence and if there is anything worthy of praise, think about these things. "(Philippians 4:6-8)

"Cast all your anxiety on him, because he cares for you. Discipline yourselves, keep alert. Like a roaring lion your adversary the devil prowls around, looking for someone to devour. Resist him, steadfast in your faith . . . And after you have suffered for a little while, the God of all grace, who has called you to his eternal glory in Christ, will himself restore, support, strengthen, and establish you." (1 Peter 5: 7-10)

"Come to me, all you who are weary and burdened, and I will give you rest. Take my yoke upon you and learn from me, for I am gentle and humble in heart, and you will find rest for your souls. For my yoke is easy and my burden is light. "(Matthew 11: 28-31)

" ..though now for a little while, if necessary, you have been grieved by various trials, so that the tested genuineness of your faith more precious than gold that perishes though it is tested by fire may be found to result in praise and glory and honor at the revelation of Jesus Christ. "(1 Peter 1:6-7)

"Be strong and courageous. Do not fear or be in dread of them, for it is the LORD your God who goes with you. He will not leave you or forsake you." (Duet. 31:6)

"The tie which links mother and child
is of such pure and immaculate strength
as to be never violated."

–Washington Irving

Index

Resources for Success

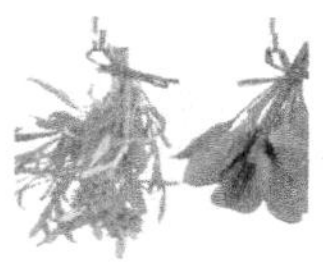

There is only one pretty child in the world and every mother has it.

-Chinese Proverb

For you [God] formed my inward parts;
you knitted me together
in my mother's womb.
I praise you, for I am fearfully
and wonderfully made.
Wonderful are your works;
my soul knows it very well.
My frame was not hidden from you,
when I was being made in secret,
intricately woven in the depths of the earth.
Your eyes saw my unformed substance;
in your book were written,
every one of them,
the days that were formed for me,
when as yet there was none of them.

– Psalm 139:13-16 ESV

NASA's Discovery about Nausea Relief

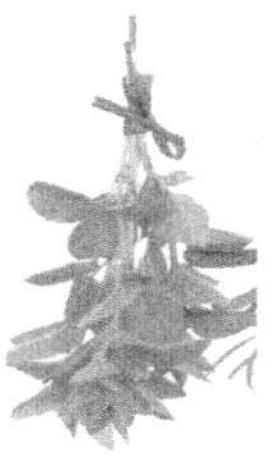

by Kevin Shaw
M.S., University North Dakota, Space Studies

"Life is not easy for any of us. But what of that?
We must have perseverance and above all confidence...
We must believe that we are gifted for something
and that this thing must be attained."

—Marie Curie

NASA has studied for years the effects of micro gravity on astronauts. During the last 50 years of space flight, close to 75% of all astronauts experience space motion sickness (SMS) to some degree while in space.

After my studies in obtaining my masters' degree in space science, I noticed that the strategies NASA used to relieve SMS could also be put to use with women battling morning sickness.

Let's start with a term called homeostasis. This is a term scientists use to describe your body's proper "balanced" state. When a woman becomes pregnant, her body no longer is in the homeostatic state that she was in prior. Her body's balance has been disrupted in areas involving: temperature, hormones, blood pH, water, potassium, etc. A change similar to an astronaut who now finds himself, about an hour after take-off, in a zero gravity environment battling his body's shift from its homeostatic state.

During the first trimester of pregnancy, a woman's body shifts from a prior homeostatic state. She now finds herself suddenly out of balance. She will suffer while her body tries to re-establish a homeostasis balance through bodily biofeedback. Biofeedback is basically the way our body's systems "talk" to themselves by increasing or decreasing secretions, etc. to bring about a balanced state.

So, what changes occur when your homeostasis has been altered ? First, your senses become more acute. They become highly sensitive. Problems with sensory input accentuate as a 'sensory mis-match' between your visual vs. vestibular regions occur. Basically, what your eyes are telling your brain is different from what ears are telling it. To complicate matters more, your motion center is located near the poison center in your brain, therefore, this proximity affects vomiting.

Also, your stomach experiences new abdominal pressures. In space, astronauts experience a head-ward fluid shift of blood. I believe, though never confirmed, that there are also fluid shifts that occur in the pregnant mom within her abdominal region that produces the nauseated response. This response, I believe, is akin to a runner who exerts himself so much in a workout that afterwards he feels like throwing up. Why ? Because a sudden blood shift away from his abdominal region towards his legs causes an onset of nausea and vomiting.

Up in space, astronauts are on immediate lookout to see when a partner loses their smile. That is the first sign of SMS onset. This makes sense. No one feels like smiling when they feel like vomiting. Next, a warm/flush feeling begins to develop, most notably in their head region. After that stage is vomiting. Interesting, astronauts in space do not feel nausea. They go right from feeling warm to vomiting, many times without warning.

What are some do's and don'ts that NASA suggests for its astronauts that you can experiment with for your morning sickness.

What Can Make Nausea Worse; "4 Do Not's"

1. Do not lie down on your back: This amplifies the sensory mismatch between your eyes and ears. You wouldn't want to lie down on your back on a rocky boat in rough waters.

2. Do not make quick body/head movements: This creates sensory-overload. Remember, your motion center is a neighbor with your poison center in the brain. Don't disturb your neighbor.

3. Do not move your head in an "Look up, Look down" plane: This causes a motion balance problem.

4. Do not have excessive visual, auditory, smells, touch, taste. Sensations: Any sensory input can trigger the nauseated/vomiting response. Even thinking about certain smells or tastes can trigger it.

What Can Help Relieve Nausea; "8 Do's"

1. Do keep your head still: This will keep your eyes and ears in better synch. Don't want the "spins".

2. Do hold on during the "Red-Zone": Vomiting episodes occur in 20-second bouts. Hang on for those 20 seconds, and the sensation may subside until the next wave hits.

3. Do use fresh, cool air: A good answer to the warm, flush feeling one gets when battling nausea.

4. Do "anchor" your feet against a wall or bed frame: Give your feet a solid foot brace, even when lying down. This will create a balanced sensation for the eyes and ears.

5. Do use dim, indirect lighting: Bright lights can cause visual- overload, and annoy you emotionally. It's similar to getting awakened in the middle of the
night when someone turns the lights on.

6. Do focus on horizontal cues when "sitting upright": Your house/room is filled with horizontal lines – focus on them. This will provide your eyes & ears with a balanced orientation. Similar, to the seasickness advice to focus on the horizon.

7. Do focus on the vertical cues when "lying down": Opposite of sitting upright. Since you're now horizontal, then focus on the vertical lines in your house/room to give you a virtual horizontal orientation/alignment.

8. Do use sensory aids that block out stimuli: Try using ear plugs, nose plugs, and eye shades to limit sensory over- stimulation.

Home Management for Challenging Days

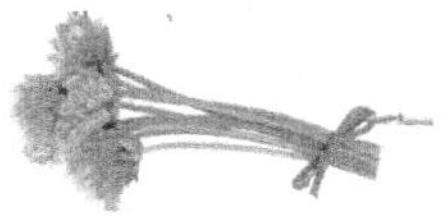

"A good laugh and a long sleep are the best cures."

~Irish Proverb

I remember my mother's prayers
and they have always followed me.
They have clung to me all my life.

–Abraham Lincoln

Managing your family and home from the bedroom, favorite chair, or couch, can be difficult. But, I want to encourage you that your family will respond resiliently to these difficult times for you! Keep a positive outlook! The needs and requirements of each family can be diverse according to the ages of your children, family dynamics and your personal tolerance levels. I'm sharing some tips we've used in our home to be able to work through common challenges until the nausea lessens. These suggestions cover a wide range of issues we faced each day (food, cleaning, play time,....). The following are tips that I found helpful from my experiences:

Meals

Frozen Meals.

It's too bad that the one area that would be nice for you to avoid right now, is so important to everyone else! Just the thought of food might make you feel queasy. If anyone ever asks what they can do for you, this is one thing to tell them- **freezer meals.** Allow a friend to solicit and organize meals from others. When I was expecting my sixth child a young lady organized a work day on my behalf. She invited over several other ladies who spent one whole day making meals for our freezer. I ended up with 20 meals! I can't express my gratitude enough on how wonderful this was for me when I needed it!

A social group may be interested in meeting your needs, or a local church.

Buy frozen meals from the store. The healthiest variety that you can purchase, within your budget.

When you do not have the energy, ability or the stomach to handle meals on a need-to-eat-now basis, pre-planning can go a long way. A good stash of 10-20 meals (at least) can be invaluable for you and your family. Your hard work beforehand can insure less work in the kitchen later on.

Crock Pot Meals.

If your mornings are usually not the best time to chop, dice and throw things into the crock pot, then do your prepping in the late afternoon, or before you go to bed. If the smell emanating from the crock pot would be hazardous for your nose, plug it in outside, or somewhere else out of your "smell zone".

Some sample meals and comfort foods: Chicken/ginger broth with chopped vegetables, Minestrone, Beef and Barley, Chicken Noodle, Beef Stew, Potato Soup or Split Pea Soup.

-Buy canned soup and keep it on warm in the crock pot.

-Reheat already prepared foods so that they will be available to you and your family at a moment's notice. Almost anything can be kept warm for your family until they are ready to sit down and eat.

Packaged Foods

These foods are readily available, portable, and can be kid friendly, too. There are increasingly more healthy choices offered. Maintaining healthy food choices and eating habits will best sustain everyone,. But, if you can't, just do the best you can. People survive almost anything!

Some foods that even our youngest could handle on their own:

Breakfast:

Cold cereals

Instant Oatmeal (my kids have eaten this with cold water), Or, cook oatmeal In the rice cooker.

Toast

Eggo's (plain, no messy syrup) or premade waffles that had been frozen

Fruit leather, or fruit

Granola Bars

Yogurt

Lunch:

-Cold Sandwiches (peanut butter/jelly, deli slices)

-Crackers with pre-sliced cheese with pre-made Vegetable/fruit trays

-Leftovers from other meals

Dinner:

-Any frozen meal that can be put in the microwave.

-Swap out breakfast and lunch dishes for dinner. (Pizza for breakfast. Cereal for dinner).

-Buy take-out in larger quantities than you need, and freeze the rest for another time.

Snacks:

-Animal crackers, graham crackers, fruit juice popsicles, pre-cut fruits and vegetables, dried fruit,.....

-Remember not to worry if all food groups are not being covered in a day or that no one is getting 3 course meals. Your family isn't going to starve from lack of variety and food choices. My family rebounded wonderfully! It's just for a season!!

-Provide a whole food vitamin or herbal supplement. (JuicePlus.com)

-At mega-stores like Costco, Sam's Club, and Smart n Final you can find many choices of bulk, easy to fix food items. Have someone get you all the food you will need for the month. Tell them your budget, and some general guidelines, and then let them do the legwork for you.

Simplify Meals

Keep your menus simple. Who said cold cereal is only for breakfast, and you can't eat dinner in the morning? Whatever works for you now supersedes all previous cultural food protocols.

Sometimes we planned meals for a week at a time, then duplicated that week throughout the month. (e.g. Every Tuesday, breakfast is Oatmeal.)

Activities for kids...

Videos

During the day it can be difficult to play with your young ones when you feel tired and/or nauseous. These are some ideas on what has worked for us:

Videos. Educational, Singing,... These can be lifesavers. Find top quality, character driven, media programs. Most videos marketed for children are silly. Redeem their time by showing character building, wholesome videos. (Hide 'em in Your Heart Vol. 1by Steve Green). Cbd.com.

Activity Baskets

Put together a basket, bin, or tub of craft starters. You don't have to lead the project., just gather a lot of fun things in one place to spark your child's imagination. If you are unable, have someone else do this. Kid safe, friendly art tools that would excite your child's creativity. Some examples are: felt, Elmer's glue, construction paper, kid friendly scissors, craft "eyes", crayons, washable markers, stickers, chalk, pipe cleaners, play-doh. Dollar stores offer some variety in crafts. Peruse a craft aisle. There is always something new and fun for kids to do. Have your children create crafts to give to others.

Door Time

Choose a room that is safe for your child to play in. Give them lots of fun things to do. Lay in front of the door inside this room. Now your younger child cannot escape, they have been provided with some fun things to do. And you can close your eyes for a few minutes, and get some needed rest.

In-Home Baby sitter

You don't have to leave to have a baby-sitter come in. This trusted person can distract and play with your little ones while you rest.

Read

If you can, read out loud to your children. Find a good book that you can all enjoy. Especially one that you can get "lost" in; a can't-put-down–until-I–know-what-happens-next, kind of book. Or, have everyone listen to an audio book.

Games

Play games that don't involve a lot of movement on your part. Some examples: I spy, Name an animal for every letter of the alphabet, … Have board games available. And, puzzles you can work on together.

Communication

When you are nauseous, communication can be tough. Here are ideas that can help: Put a whiteboard/chalkboard/boogieboard near you. Write your needs on it. "Bring me Ice, ASAP," "Let me sleep a little bit longer." "Check on me every 15 minutes." etc. (myboogieboard.com/na/)

Bells, Whistles & Cell Phones

When your strength is gone. Or you just cannot yell out loud enough to be heard, then you can use bells or a whistle to communicate much louder than your voice can carry. Use your cell phone to call your house phone or email/text/call someone. Invest in an intercom. Kids have fun with walkie talkies.

House Maintenance

Laundry

Laundry- If you *can* get a load done, don't bother folding it. The laundry basket makes a nice holding tank for clean clothes. Conserve (re-use) towels for smaller overall loads.

Quick Cleans

Please don't expect your house to look perfect. You are living there and above that, not feeling well; it's OK for your house to reflect that. Your house is not a top priority right now. However, too much mess can be depressing, so, have a big tub and have your family do "quick cleans" throughout the day collecting things to sort through later. You may want to make a game out of this for your children – "For the next 2 minutes, find 10 things on the floor that do not belong there, and toss it in the tub. Let's see who can find the most things!"

Outside Help

Accept the offers of others to do maid service!

Consider hiring a maid for just some rooms like bathrooms and/or kitchens, for a short time.

Just One Room

The house could be messy, but it was nice to have one room always kept orderly, as a sanctuary. Being around a mess all day isn't good for your well being either. You will feel better being in a room that is tidy. In addition, if possible, have something in that room that is pretty to look at, (flowers, scenic window view) this can be a small inspiration.

Set Small Goals

Set small housekeeping or family goals. Even if you accomplish just one thing on your list. (ex. wipe down counters) you have done something. Now go back and rest.

If you need distractions from nausea, set small goals, then keep going down your list as much as you are able. By breaking down the goals into smaller more achievable options, the accomplishment will seem greater and the satisfaction higher.

Buddies

Kids can help each other. We found it helpful to team up the children into buddies. The older child is responsible to watch over the younger one. Even when our youngest buddies were four and two. They had fun with this concept. The older one delighted in the responsibility, and the younger one naturally looked up to the older sibling and liked the special attention.

Some examples of what buddies can do for each other are:

Help brush teeth.

Help pick up toys.

Get a drink of water.

Color with each other.

Help serve meals.

Sing together.

Read to the younger one.

Make a fort. (A blanket over the dining room table).

Don't forget to designate someone as your buddy. This person will check on you throughout the day and bring you the things that you need.

Loving Your Family When.....

...you're exhausted, irritable, frustrated, depressed, hurting, and sick.... Continue to communicate tokens of love!

Plan on communicating extra love to those around you when you're feeling this way.

Ideas:

~ Write little love notes.

~Be the first to give a big smile.

~Express appreciation for the little things.

~ Ask your loved one to tell you about their day, or their thoughts.

~ Compliment for the slightest of favors.

~ Say "I love you" frequently.

~Lots of hugs.

"There is no remedy for love but to love more."

– Henry David Thoreau

Some Homeschool Tips for the "Challenging Days."

You don't homeschool? My husband likes to say, "Everyone homeschools...each parent just decides how much and how often they do it." All learning begins at home!

When you need to keep your child busy with productive work:

- Have workbook based activities.
- Assign research projects.
- Show educational videos. (Youtube.com as lots of videos on, "How do they do that?" for an interesting way to learn about how things are made.
- Co-op with friends for lessons.
- Set new, personal learning goals and then reward accomplishments.
- Continue to encourage self-motivation.
- Daily Bible Quiz: DailyBibleLessons.com
- Character + Handwriting practice = Success CharacterWritingWorksheets.com
- Christian resources for books, videos, etc.: Cbd.com
- Intelligent things for kids to do: Timberdoodle.com
- Science ideas and labs: HomeScienceTools.com
- Enjoy this Family Music Band together: www.josties.com/

References/Sources

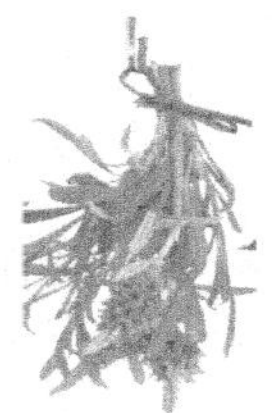

"Every tomorrow has two handles.
We can take hold of it with the handle of anxiety
or the handle of faith."
-Henry Ward Beecher

Books about Morning Sickness

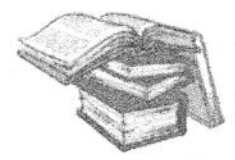

Real life experiences or researched books of women who have experienced nausea in varying degrees.

The Good, The Bad, The Blessing by Camilia Harris-Butler. www.thegoodthebadtheblessing.com

Body Mutiny by Jenna Schmitt. www.extrememorningsickness.com

No More Morning Sickness- A Survival Guide for Pregnant Women

Managing Your Morning Sickness by Miriam Erick. www.morningsickness.net

The Morning Sickness Companion by Elizabeth Kaledin

The Proving Grounds by Babara Mangini

Morning Sickness 24/7 by Tabby L. Silcott

Natural Remedy Books

The Naturally Healthy Pregnancy by Shonda Parker

Prescription for Herbal Healing by Phyllis A. Balch

Nutrition for a Healthy Pregnancy: The Complete Guide to Eating Before, During and After Your Pregnancy by Elizabeth Somer

Herbs for A Healthy Pregnancy by Penelope Ody

Discovering Homeopathy: Medicine for the 21st Century by Dana Ullman

Eating for Pregnancy: An Essential Guide to Nutrition with Recipes for the WholeFamily by Catherine Cheremeteff Jones, Rose Ann Hudson

The Wise Woman Herbal For The Childbearing Years by Susan Weed [We placed a big sticker on the cover to hide the nude picture.]

Nourishing Traditions by Sally Fallon - Food preparation for optimal nutrition.

Sites to Find Support

www.motherrisk.com - An incredibly friendly staff that will answer all your questions about drugs and medications in pregnancy.

www.helpher.org - The best place to get the latest research on hyperemsis and find a friend who is experiencing it also.

www.sosmorningsickness.com - Helpline 1-800-436- 8477

www.stpatrickscottsdale.org. - If you live in AZ, founded by Jenna Schmitt, author of Body Mutiny.

Weston Price Foundation. - Healthy eating.

Morning Sickness Forums/Blogs

http://forums.llli.org – La Leche League Forum

www.mothering.com

www.welltellme.com

http://forums.helpher.org/ – HG Research Organization

http://www.i-am-pregnant.com - HG Forum

www.cafemom.com

http://momys.com/

http://www.whattoexpect.com/forum

Other Sources Used:

http://en.wikipedia.org/wiki/Morning_sickness

http://en.wikipedia.org/wiki/Hyperemesis_gravidarum

http://whfoods.org/

Products

CoconutTraditions.com – Tropical Traditions products go above and beyond organic! Essential oils, grass fed beef, free range eggs, etc. TT tests all products for glyphosate.

youngliving.com – Essential oils

doterrra.com – Essential oils

frontierherb.com

bulkherbstore.com

mymorningsickness.com – General Store

morningwell.co.uk/ – Audio CD

morningsicknesshelp.com – Variety of products

mountainmeadowherbs.com - Morning Sickness Balm

karenhurd.com - Beans help with nausea

hpathy.com – Find a Homeopathic Doctor in your area

trilighttherbs.com

http://drkowalski.stores.yahoo.net/en500mg90son.html - Entrox

traditionalmedicinals.com

gardenoflife.com/ - Probiotics * Vitamins

wellnessmama.com - Health blog, homemade ginger ale

collegefarmorganic.com/ - Organic candy

morningchicnessbags.com – Tara Ramos stylish bags,....just in case.

vitacost.com – Well priced vitamins and supplements

babybirthandbeyond.com - Birth supplies, etc.

GNOFGLINS.com – Traditional food cooking.

Favorite Christian Resources:

aboverubies.org - Ministry to Moms

rzim.org – Apologetics

wholeheart.org – Exists to equip and encourage Moms

ElizabethGeorge.com – My favorite Christian author

A Silver Lining in the Nausea Cloud?

Morning Sickness Has Been Tied to Lower Breast Cancer Risk:

http://www.buffalo.edu/news/8704

"Faith is deliberate confidence in the character of God whose ways you may not understand at the time."

-Oswald Chambers

If you need encouragement, information, prayer and support while you joyfully celebrate this special time in your life, contact me.

Tell me about your experience and how you are feeling.

wendy@mymorningsickness.com

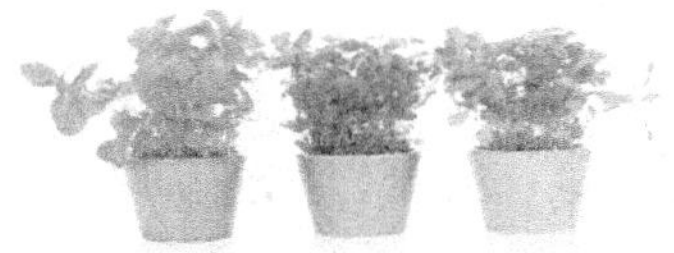

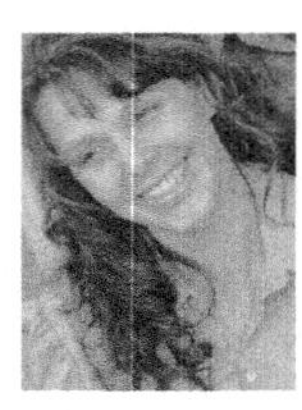

About the Author

In my first pregnancy, I was diagnosed with hyperemesis gravidarum (severe morning sickness). This was a catalyst to relentlessly search for a remedy to find relief. And, then to discover a way to help other women who were also experiencing morning sickness - in all its varying degrees. I hosted teleconferences with expert "morning sickness" authors to share and support the moms who were dealing with their nausea. And, created the site: MyMorningSickness.com to help provide information and support the blessed pregnant Mamas. My husband of 23 years, Kevin, and I live near Yosemite National Park, with our 10 children.

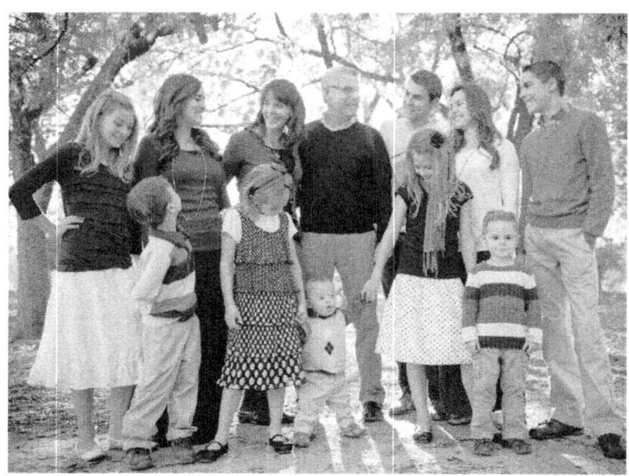

Kevin & Wendy Shaw, Chase, Holly, Macy, Justus,

Elley, Amy, Lilly, Peter and Daniel & Joshua

Other Books by this Author:

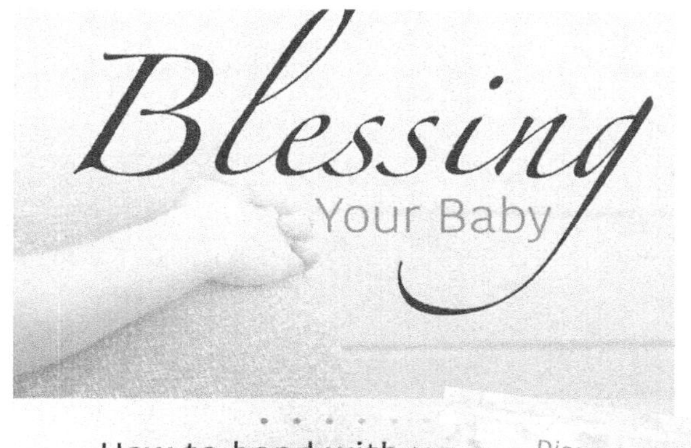

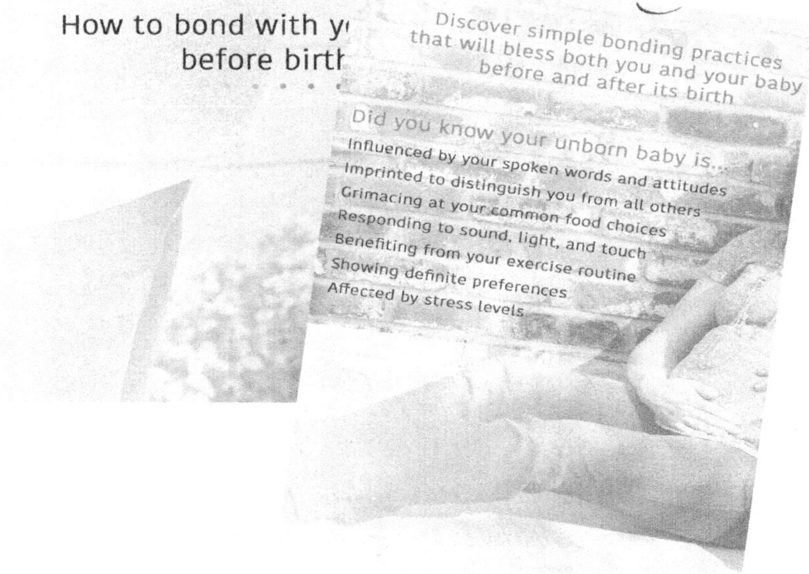

Blessing Your Baby by Wendy Shaw - Babies in the womb are already responding to their outside environment. Moms can bond with their baby right now, before its born! An important and fun read for all pregnant moms.

Order from MyMorningSickness.com or Amazon.com

Psalm 127:3-5

Behold, children are a heritage from the Lord,
the fruit of the womb a reward.
Like arrows in the hand of a warrior
are the children of one's youth.
Blessed is the man
who fills his quiver with them!
He shall not be put to shame
when he speaks with his enemies in the gate.

Made in the USA
Coppell, TX
03 January 2020

13973991R00069